The Resilient Mind
JOURNAL

Robert Armstrong
Library User Group

The Resilient Mind Journal — Part 1: Laying the Foundation

Part 1 of The Resilient Mind Journal is about rebuilding strength from the inside out.
Before growth, before clarity, before momentum—resilience must be established. This first section is designed to help you slow down, reflect honestly, and reconnect with the core of who you are beneath stress, setbacks, and expectations.

Life has a way of hardening the mind through pressure, disappointment, and constant demands. Over time, unprocessed thoughts and emotions create mental fatigue, self-doubt, and emotional overload. Part 1 exists to interrupt that cycle.

This section focuses on awareness, grounding, and emotional reset. The prompts gently guide you to examine what you've been carrying, what has shaped you, and what deserves to be released. There is no pressure to "fix" anything here—only space to observe, understand, and begin again with clarity.

Why Part 1 Is So Important

Resilience isn't about ignoring pain or pushing through at all costs. True resilience is built when you acknowledge your inner experience without judgment. Part 1 lays the groundwork for that process by helping you:

Recognize emotional patterns that no longer serve you

Identify sources of stress, fear, or mental exhaustion

Reconnect with your inner voice and sense of control

Create a calm, stable mental foundation for future growth

Without this foundation, personal growth efforts often feel forced or temporary. Part 1 ensures that everything that follows is rooted in self-awareness and emotional honesty.

The Power of Using This Journal Consistently

Using The Resilient Mind Journal regularly—especially in Part 1—creates a quiet but powerful shift. Writing engages the brain differently than thinking alone. It slows racing thoughts, reduces emotional intensity, and brings clarity to complex feelings. Over time, this practice strengthens emotional regulation, improves self-trust, and restores a sense of inner balance.

Consistency matters more than perfection. Even a few minutes a day can:

Reduce mental overwhelm

Improve emotional resilience

Increase self-understanding

Build confidence in your ability to handle challenges

This journal is not meant to be rushed. It is meant to be returned to—day after day—as a steady companion during moments of reflection, recovery, and renewal.

Part 1 is the beginning of resilience—not as a concept, but as a lived experience.
By committing to this section, you are choosing to strengthen your mind, honor your journey, and prepare yourself for growth that lasts.

Copyright 2025 by Library User Group

All rights reserved. No part of this publication may be reproduced,
distributed, or transmitted in any from or by any means, including photocopying, recording or other electronic or mechanical methods,
without the prior written permisiion of the publisher, except in the
noncommercial users permitted by copyright law. For permission requests, please email the publisher with the subject line "Attention:
 Permissions Coordinator" at: Email: contact#libraryusergroup.com

Ordering Information:
Quantity Sales: Special discounts are available for quantity purchases by corporations, assouciations, and others.
For details, contact the publisher at:
:Email: contact#libraryusergroup.com

For orders from U.S. trade bookstores and wholesalers, please contact contact your distribution channel.

The Resilient Mind Journal 1

ISBN: 978-1-63553-030-8

Diaries & Journals

FIRST EDITION

Arriving Here

Begin by writing what brought you to this journal—whether it was curiosity, exhaustion, change, healing, or a quiet need for clarity. There is no right reason to be here. Simply acknowledge the path that led you to open these pages.

A Moment to Pause

Take a brief pause to breathe and write whatever is present in your mind or body right now, without judgment, expectation, or the need to fix anything.

_____

_____

_____

_____

_____

_____

_____

_____

_____

_____

_____

_____

_____

_____

What I'm Carrying Right Now

Write about the thoughts, emotions, responsibilities, or worries you've been holding onto lately, acknowledging them honestly without trying to judge, minimize, or resolve them.

_____

_____

_____

_____

_____

_____

_____

_____

_____

_____

_____

_____

_____

_____

Naming the Weight

Put words to the specific feelings, pressures, or burdens that feel heaviest right now, giving them a name so they no longer remain unspoken or undefined.

Where My Energy Goes

Reflect on what people, tasks, or thoughts have been consuming most of your energy lately and how that affects your mood, focus, and well-being.

When Life Feels Heavy

Describe moments or situations when life feels overwhelming and what thoughts or emotions tend to surface during those times.

_____

_____

_____

_____

_____

_____

_____

_____

_____

_____

_____

_____

_____

_____

_____

What Drains Me Most

Identify the people, situations, habits, or thoughts that leave you feeling most depleted and note how they impact your energy or mindset.

_____

_____

_____

_____

_____

_____

_____

_____

_____

_____

_____

_____

_____

What Still Holds Me Up

Write about the supports, strengths, habits, or people that continue to steady you, even during difficult or exhausting times.

The Space Between Thoughts

Notice and describe the quiet moments between your thoughts, focusing on how it feels when your mind slows, even briefly.

Breathing Room

Write about anything that gives you a sense of relief, openness, or calm, and how creating more space—mentally or emotionally—might help you right now.

What I Avoid Thinking About

Gently explore the thoughts or topics you tend to push aside or distract yourself from, noting why they feel difficult to face without forcing yourself to go deeper than you're ready for.

What I Need to Acknowledge

Write honestly about something you know deserves your attention right now, even if it feels uncomfortable or easy to overlook.

The Story I Tell Myself

Describe the narrative you often repeat in your mind about yourself or your situation, noticing how it shapes your feelings and reactions.

Where That Story Began

Reflect on when and where that personal story first took shape, considering the experiences or moments that may have influenced it.

_____

_____

_____

_____

_____

_____

_____

_____

_____

_____

_____

_____

_____

_____

What I've Learned About Surviving

Write about the lessons, coping skills, or inner strengths you've developed through difficult experiences and how they've helped you keep going.

Strength I Forgot I Had

Recall a time when you showed strength you may have overlooked or forgotten, and reflect on what that says about you now.

Moments That Shaped Me

Write about specific experiences—big or small—that have significantly influenced who you are today and how you see the world.

What I've Outgrown

Reflect on beliefs, habits, roles, or relationships that no longer fit who you are becoming and how releasing them might create space for growth.

_____

_____

_____

_____

_____

_____

_____

_____

_____

_____

_____

_____

_____

_____

Letting Go (Without Forcing It)

Write about something you're not ready to release yet, while gently exploring what it might feel like to loosen your grip without pressure or urgency.

Emotional Clutter

Identify lingering emotions, unresolved thoughts, or mental noise that feel crowded or overwhelming, simply naming them without needing to clear them away yet.

_____

_____

_____

_____

_____

_____

_____

_____

_____

_____

_____

_____

_____

Where I Feel Safe

Write about places, people, routines, or inner feelings that give you a sense of safety and comfort, and what makes them grounding for you.

___

___

___

___

___

___

___

___

___

___

___

___

___

Where I Don't

Reflect on situations, environments, or relationships where you feel uneasy or unprotected, noticing what signals your discomfort without self-judgment.

_____

_____

_____

_____

_____

_____

_____

_____

_____

_____

_____

_____

_____

_____

Listening to My Inner Voice

Write about what your inner voice has been trying to tell you lately and whether you've been listening, ignoring it, or questioning it.

What My Body Is Telling Me

Notice physical sensations, tension, or fatigue you've been experiencing and reflect on what your body might be communicating about your needs.

_____

_____

_____

_____

_____

_____

_____

_____

_____

_____

_____

_____

_____

_____

_____

Signals I've Ignored

Write about emotional or physical warning signs you've noticed but pushed aside, and what they may be asking for now.

_____

_____

_____

_____

_____

_____

_____

_____

_____

_____

_____

_____

_____

The Cost of Holding It In
Reflect on how suppressing your thoughts or emotions has affected your well-being, relationships, or sense of self.

Permission to Rest

Write about what rest truly means to you right now and what might change if you allowed yourself to take it without guilt.

What Calm Feels Like

Describe how calm shows up for you—physically, emotionally, or mentally—and what helps you recognize it when it appears.

_____

_____

_____

_____

_____

_____

_____

_____

_____

_____

_____

_____

_____

_____

Creating Mental Space

Write about ways you can reduce mental clutter or distractions to create more openness and clarity in your thoughts.

_____

_____

_____

_____

_____

_____

_____

_____

_____

_____

_____

_____

_____

_____

My Definition of Balance
Reflect on what balance truly means in your life right now and how it differs from what you think it *should* look like.

What I Can Control Today

Write about the small, manageable choices or actions within your control today, focusing on what feels supportive rather than overwhelming.

What I Can Release

Reflect on a thought, expectation, or pressure you're ready to loosen or let go of, even if only a little, to create more ease.

_____

_____

_____

_____

_____

_____

_____

_____

_____

_____

_____

_____

_____

_____

Patterns I'm Ready to Notice

Write about recurring thoughts, behaviors, or emotional reactions you're beginning to see more clearly and are open to understanding.

Responding Instead of Reacting

Reflect on situations where you tend to react automatically and explore how pausing might help you respond with more intention.

Where I Need Gentleness

Write about areas of your life or parts of yourself that could benefit from more compassion, patience, or softness right now.

_____

_____

_____

_____

_____

_____

_____

_____

_____

_____

_____

_____

_____

Boundaries I'm Beginning to See

Reflect on limits you're starting to recognize around your time, energy, or emotions and what honoring them might look like.

_____

_____

_____

_____

_____

_____

_____

_____

_____

_____

_____

_____

_____

_____

Rebuilding Trust With Myself

Write about ways you can begin to trust your own decisions, feelings, or instincts again, especially after times when that trust was shaken.

What Resilience Means to Me

Reflect on your personal understanding of resilience and how it shows up in your life beyond simply pushing through challenges.

_____

_____

_____

_____

_____

_____

_____

_____

_____

_____

_____

_____

_____

_____

Small Wins That Matter

Write about recent small accomplishments or moments of progress that deserve recognition, even if they seem minor.

Progress Without Pressure

Reflect on how you can move forward at your own pace without forcing growth or measuring yourself against expectations.

Who I Am Beneath the Stress
Write about the parts of yourself that exist beyond pressure and responsibility, reconnecting with who you are when stress fades.

_____

_____

_____

_____

_____

_____

_____

_____

_____

_____

_____

_____

_____

What Still Brings Me Peace

Reflect on people, activities, or moments that continue to bring you a sense of peace, even during difficult times.

_____

_____

_____

_____

_____

_____

_____

_____

_____

_____

_____

_____

_____

Strength in Stillness

Write about how slowing down or being still has helped you regain clarity, balance, or inner strength.

Allowing Imperfection

Reflect on where you can give yourself permission to be imperfect and how that acceptance might ease pressure or self-criticism.

The Power of Showing Up

Write about times when simply being present or trying, even imperfectly, made a meaningful difference.

One Thought I Can Reframe

Write down a recurring thought that feels limiting or heavy and explore a gentler, more supportive way to look at it.

Grounded, Not Perfect

Reflect on what helps you feel steady and rooted, even when everything isn't finished, fixed, or ideal.

Today's Emotional Check-In
Briefly note how you're feeling emotionally right now, naming your feelings honestly without trying to change them.

_____

_____

_____

_____

_____

_____

_____

_____

_____

_____

_____

_____

_____

_____

What I Want to Carry Forward

Write about the insights, feelings, or strengths you want to take with you as you continue moving forward.

_____

_____

_____

_____

_____

_____

_____

_____

_____

_____

_____

_____

_____

Laying the Foundation

Reflect on what you are intentionally building within yourself right now and the steady, supportive steps that will help it take root.

Settling Into the Page

Write about how it feels to slow down, be present, and ease into this moment with the page in front of you.

Checking In With Myself
Take an honest snapshot of your current thoughts, emotions, and energy level, noting how you're truly doing right now.

What Feels Unfinished

Write about thoughts, emotions, or situations that still feel unresolved and gently acknowledge them without needing closure yet.

___

___

___

___

___

___

___

___

___

___

___

___

___

The Quiet Beneath the Noise
Notice and describe the calm or clarity that exists underneath busy thoughts, even if it feels faint or brief.

What I Need More Of

Reflect on qualities, experiences, or support you wish you had more of right now and why they feel important.

___

___

___

___

___

___

___

___

___

___

___

___

___

Todays thoughts

Write a brief, honest snapshot of the thoughts that have been most present in your mind today, without filtering or judging them.

_____

_____

_____

_____

_____

_____

_____

_____

_____

_____

_____

_____

_____

A Thought Worth Sitting With

Write down a single thought that keeps returning and take time to explore it gently instead of pushing it away.

Where My Attention Drifts

Notice where your focus tends to wander during the day and reflect on what those distractions might be signaling.

What Feels Steady

Write about the people, routines, beliefs, or inner qualities that give you a sense of stability right now.

What Feels Uncertain
Reflect on areas of your life that feel unclear or unsettled and how that uncertainty affects you emotionally.

_____

_____

_____

_____

_____

_____

_____

_____

_____

_____

_____

_____

_____

_____

_____

Emotional Weather Today

Describe your current emotional state as if it were weather, noting its tone, intensity, and any shifts you notice.

The Pace I'm Moving At

Reflect on how fast or slow you've been moving lately and whether that pace feels supportive or exhausting.

What I'm Holding Too Tightly
Write about a thought, expectation, or situation you may be gripping too tightly and how easing that hold could bring relief.

What I'm Afraid to Release
Gently explore something you fear letting go of and what you worry might happen if you did.

When I Feel Most Like Myself

Write about moments or activities when you feel most authentic, grounded, and connected to who you truly are.

___
___
___
___
___
___
___
___
___
___
___
___

When I Feel Disconnected

Reflect on times when you feel distant from yourself or others and what seems to contribute to that feeling.

What Helps Me Reset
Write about actions, habits, or moments that help you regain balance and clarity when you feel off track.

Signs I'm Overwhelmed

Notice and write about the emotional, mental, or physical signals that show up when you're feeling overwhelmed.

_____

_____

_____

_____

_____

_____

_____

_____

_____

_____

_____

_____

_____

Gentle Ways to Cope

Write about kind, low-pressure ways you support yourself during stress, focusing on comfort rather than fixing.

The Space I Need Right Now
Reflect on what kind of physical, emotional, or mental space would feel most supportive for you in this moment.

_____

_____

_____

_____

_____

_____

_____

_____

_____

_____

_____

_____

_____

_____

What Deserves My Energy

Write about the people, priorities, or activities that truly deserve your time and energy right now.

What Can Wait

Identify tasks, worries, or expectations that don't need your immediate attention and allow yourself to set them aside for now.

How I Speak to Myself

Reflect on the tone and language of your inner dialogue and how it influences your emotions and confidence.

A Thought I Can Soften
Write about a harsh or rigid thought you've been carrying and explore how you might gently soften it with compassion or perspective.

Where I Feel Tension

Notice where tension shows up in your body or mind and reflect on what it might be responding to.

Moments of Quiet Strength

Write about subtle moments when you showed strength without recognition or force, simply by staying present or enduring.

What I Can Simplify

Reflect on areas of your life that feel overly complicated and how simplifying them might bring relief or clarity.

Where I Need Patience

Write about situations or areas of your life that require more patience from you and what makes waiting difficult.

_____

_____

_____

_____

_____

_____

_____

_____

_____

_____

_____

_____

_____

_____

_____

Trusting the Process

Reflect on where you are being asked to trust gradual progress and uncertainty rather than immediate results.

One Step at a Time

Write about the next small, manageable step you can take without worrying about the entire journey.

What I Notice When I Slow Down
Reflect on thoughts, feelings, or details that become clearer when you intentionally slow your pace.

Giving Myself Grace

Write about how you can offer yourself kindness and understanding instead of criticism, especially in moments when things don't go as planned.

_____

_____

_____

_____

_____

_____

_____

_____

_____

_____

_____

_____

_____

What Stability Means to Me
Reflect on what stability looks and feels like in your life right now and what helps create it.

When I Feel Grounded

Write about moments, places, or practices that help you feel centered, steady, and connected to the present.

___
___
___
___
___
___
___
___
___
___
___
___
___
___
___

What Disrupts My Calm

Reflect on situations, thoughts, or behaviors that tend to disturb your sense of calm and why they have that effect.

Returning to Center

Write about what helps you realign with yourself after feeling scattered, stressed, or off balance.

Choosing Awareness

Reflect on moments when becoming more aware of your thoughts or feelings could help you respond with intention rather than habit.

Letting This Be Enough

Write about what it would feel like to accept this moment, effort, or version of yourself as sufficient without needing more.

Holding Space for Myself

Write about how you can allow yourself to feel and process your experiences with patience, compassion, and without self-judgment.

___

___

___

___

___

___

___

___

___

___

___

___

___

___

___

Beginning Without Pressure

Reflect on how you can start or continue this journey gently, without rushing, expectations, or the need to have everything figured out.

Resilience isn't about avoiding hardship—it's about learning how to rise from it.

The Resilient Mind Journal is a guided space for reflection, clarity, and emotional strength. Part 1 helps you slow down, release mental overload, and reconnect with the thoughts and experiences that shape your inner world.

Through thoughtful prompts and intentional pauses, this journal encourages self-awareness, calm, and honest reflection—without pressure or perfection. Each page is an invitation to reset your mindset, strengthen emotional balance, and begin building resilience from within.

Whether you're navigating stress, change, or personal growth, this journal meets you where you are and helps you move forward—one page at a time.

Your journey toward a stronger, clearer mind begins here.

www.ingramcontent.com/pod-product-compliance
Lightning Source LLC
Chambersburg PA
CBHW030913080526
44589CB00010B/290